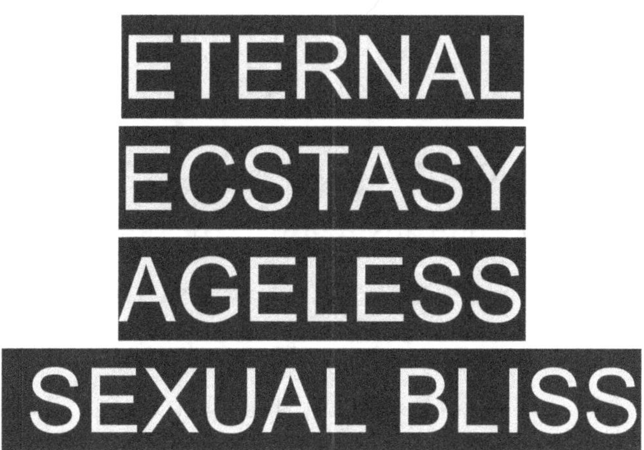

# ETERNAL ECSTASY AGELESS SEXUAL BLISS

## Unlocking the Secrets of Passionate Pleasure After 40s

By

Dora J. Boye

## Table of contents

# Introduction

In a society where youth and vitality are celebrated, the notion of ageless sexual bliss seems like an elusive dream. However, within the captivating pages of "Eternal Ecstasy: Ageless Sexual Bliss," author Dora J. Boye takes readers on a remarkable journey, unravelling the deep mysteries of passion and desire that transcend the boundaries of age. Drawing upon her own profound experience and personal triumph, Boye weaves a tapestry of sensuality, wisdom, and self-discovery that will leave readers inspired and captivated.

At the tender age of 75, when most people believe the flames of passion have long been extinguished, Dora J. Boye encountered a significant turning point in her life. She experienced a profound loss of appetite for sex, leaving her feeling disconnected from her own body and the cherished intimacy it once held. However, rather than succumbing to resignation, Boye embarked on a transformative quest to reclaim her sexual vitality, unearthing secrets that would challenge societal norms and redefine the boundaries of pleasure.

"Eternal Ecstasy: Ageless Sexual Bliss" serves as both a memoir and a guide, inviting readers into Boye's world of vulnerability, self-reflection, and empowerment. With profound candour, she shares her personal experiences, both triumphs and setbacks, offering a roadmap for individuals seeking to revitalise their own intimate lives, regardless of age or circumstance. Boye's writing radiates with warmth, compassion, and a deep understanding of the complexities of human sexuality. Through her vivid storytelling, she explores the psychological, emotional, and physical dimensions of sex, guiding readers towards a renewed sense of self-awareness and the unearthing of hidden desires. Her words serve as a catalyst for embracing one's own unique sensual journey, encouraging readers to embrace their bodies, explore their fantasies, and connect with their partners on a deeper, more profound level.

Within the pages of "Eternal Ecstasy: Ageless Sexual Bliss," Dora J. Boye presents a revolutionary approach to intimacy, challenging societal misconceptions about ageing and pleasure. Her story is an invitation to break free from the limitations imposed by time and societal expectations, opening up a world of infinite possibility, where sexual bliss knows no bounds. As readers immerse themselves in Boye's remarkable narrative, they will discover that true ecstasy transcends age, and that within each individual lies the potential for a lifetime of fulfilment and passionate connection.

Prepare to be captivated, enlightened, and inspired as you embark on this unforgettable journey with Dora J. Boye in "Eternal Ecstasy: Ageless Sexual Bliss."

# Book description

Are you ready to unlock the secrets to eternal pleasure and experience ageless sexual bliss like never before? In "Eternal Ecstasy: Ageless Sexual Bliss," Renowned intimacy expert, takes you on an exhilarating journey through the depths of passion, revealing ancient wisdom and groundbreaking techniques that will forever transform your sexual experiences.

Do you long to reignite the flames of desire and achieve a level of intimacy that transcends time? Driven by her insatiable curiosity and unyielding commitment to unravel the mysteries of pleasure, Dora J. Boye has travelled the globe, unearthing forgotten techniques from ancient civilizations and delving into cutting-edge research to present you with a treasure trove of sexual knowledge.

Within the pages of this captivating guide, you will discover:

How to harness your own innate sensual power to unlock the gates of ecstasy.

Secrets to rejuvenating your sexual energy and experiencing ageless desire.

Ancient tantric practices that will ignite your passion and deepen your connection with your partner.

Innovative techniques to overcome common obstacles and achieve mind-blowing orgasms.

Strategies to maintain sexual vitality and experience pleasure at any age.

Prepare to be captivated by my unparalleled expertise and her ability to demystify complex concepts, making them accessible to anyone seeking profound sexual fulfilment. Each page of "Eternal Ecstasy" is filled with thought-provoking insights, practical exercises, and intimate stories of individuals who have embarked on this transformative journey to eternal bliss.

Now is the time to reclaim your sexual power and embark on an extraordinary adventure of pleasure that transcends the limitations of time. Don't miss your chance to own this extraordinary guide that will revolutionise your sexual experiences and leave you craving for more.

Unlock the secrets of eternal ecstasy and experience ageless sexual bliss like never before. Get your copy of "Eternal Ecstasy: Ageless Sexual Bliss" now and embark on a journey that will forever change the way you perceive pleasure. Act quickly, for your time to experience this profound transformation is now!

**Chapter One**

# MEANING OF POLYCYSTIC OVARIAN SYNDROME (PCOS)

In the pursuit of eternal ecstasy and ageless sexual bliss, it is crucial to understand the various factors that can affect women's reproductive health. One such condition that significantly impacts women's lives is Polycystic Ovarian Syndrome (PCOS). This chapter aims to provide a comprehensive explanation of PCOS, its meaning, symptoms, and potential implications on sexual well-being.

Understanding Polycystic Ovarian Syndrome (PCOS):

Polycystic Ovarian Syndrome, commonly known as PCOS, is a hormonal disorder that affects women of reproductive age. It is characterised by imbalanced hormone levels, irregular menstrual cycles, and the development of small cysts on the ovaries. PCOS can have far-reaching consequences on a woman's physical, emotional, and sexual health.

Symptoms and Manifestations:

The symptoms of PCOS can vary from woman to woman and may include irregular or absent menstrual periods, excessive hair growth (hirsutism), acne, weight gain, and fertility issues. These symptoms often arise due to an overproduction of androgens, which are male hormones that women also produce in smaller amounts. The hormonal imbalances in PCOS can disrupt the regular ovulation process, leading to difficulties in conceiving.

Implications on Sexual Well-being:

PCOS can have a profound impact on a woman's sexual well-being, affecting both physical and emotional aspects of intimacy. Hormonal imbalances can lead to decreased libido, vaginal dryness, and discomfort during intercourse. The psychological effects of PCOS, such as body image concerns, mood swings, and anxiety, can also impact a woman's ability to fully engage in sexual experiences and derive pleasure.

Management and Treatment:

While PCOS is a lifelong condition, its symptoms and impact on sexual well-being can be effectively managed through various approaches. Lifestyle modifications, such as regular exercise, a balanced diet, and weight management, play a crucial role in minimising the symptoms of PCOS. Medications, such as hormonal contraceptives or insulin-sensitising agents, may be prescribed to regulate menstrual cycles, reduce androgen levels, and improve fertility.

Embracing Support and Seeking Professional Help:

Dealing with PCOS can be challenging, and women with this condition may find solace in support groups, counselling, or therapy. Sharing experiences and seeking guidance from professionals can help individuals navigate the physical and emotional aspects of PCOS and foster a healthier relationship with their bodies and sexuality.

**Foot words.**

Polycystic Ovarian Syndrome is a complex hormonal disorder that affects numerous women worldwide. By understanding the meaning of PCOS and its implications on sexual well-being, women can empower themselves to seek appropriate treatment, adopt a healthy lifestyle, and cultivate fulfilling intimate relationships. Through education, support, and effective management strategies, women can aspire to achieve eternal ecstasy and ageless sexual bliss despite the challenges posed by PCOS.

**Chapter Two**

# FACTS AND HISTORY OF PCOS

Polycystic Ovary Syndrome (PCOS) is a common hormonal disorder that affects many women worldwide. It is essential to delve into the facts and history of PCOS to better understand its impact on women's health. By gaining knowledge about this condition, you can make informed decisions when purchasing products or seeking treatments related to PCOS. In this note, we will explore the facts and history of PCOS and explain how this knowledge can empower your buying decisions.

Facts about PCOS:

Prevalence: PCOS affects approximately 5-10% of women of reproductive age globally, making it one of the most common hormonal disorders in women.

Hormonal Imbalance: PCOS is characterised by an imbalance in reproductive hormones, specifically androgens (male hormones) and insulin.

Symptoms: Common symptoms of PCOS include irregular menstrual cycles, excessive hair growth (hirsutism), acne, weight gain, and fertility issues.

Health Risks: Women with PCOS are at a higher risk of developing health conditions such as type 2 diabetes, heart disease, high blood pressure, and endometrial cancer.

Diagnosis: PCOS is diagnosed based on symptoms, medical history, physical examinations, and additional tests, such as hormone level measurements and ultrasound imaging.

Historical Context:

Discovery: PCOS was first described in 1935 by American gynaecologists Irving F. Stein, Michael L. Leventhal, and M. I. Mochizuki, who observed enlarged ovaries with cysts in women experiencing menstrual irregularities.

Evolving Understanding: Over the years, medical professionals and researchers have made significant progress in understanding PCOS. The Rotterdam Criteria, established in 2003, provided a comprehensive definition for diagnosing PCOS, considering multiple symptoms and excluding other causes.

Research Advances: Ongoing scientific research aims to uncover the underlying causes, genetic factors, and effective treatment options for PCOS. This has led to improved management strategies and a better understanding of the condition's long-term implications.

Empowering Buying Decisions:

Awareness of Symptoms: Understanding the symptoms of PCOS can help you identify products or treatments that address specific concerns. For example, if you struggle with acne or excessive hair growth, you can choose skincare products or hair removal techniques specifically formulated for PCOS-related issues.

Consultation with Healthcare Professionals: Discussing your condition and treatment options with healthcare professionals can provide valuable insights into the most suitable products or medications for managing PCOS-related symptoms.

Researching Trusted Brands: Conduct thorough research on brands that specialise in PCOS-related products. Look for companies with a history of creating reliable, evidence-based solutions to ensure you make informed purchasing decisions.

Peer Reviews and Support Communities: Engage with peer reviews and online support communities where individuals with PCOS share their experiences and recommend products or treatments that have worked for them.

**Chapter Three**

# ORIGIN OF PCOS

While the exact origin of PCOS is not fully understood, research suggests that it is likely caused by a combination of genetic, hormonal, and environmental factors. In this elaborate note, I will provide an explanation of the possible origins of PCOS.

Genetic Factors:

There is strong evidence to suggest that genetics play a significant role in the development of PCOS. Studies have shown that women with PCOS often have close relatives, such as mothers or sisters, who also have the condition. Researchers have identified several candidate genes that may contribute to PCOS, although no single gene has been identified as the sole cause.

Hormonal Imbalances:

Hormonal imbalances, particularly involving insulin and androgens, are commonly observed in women with PCOS. Insulin resistance, a condition in which the body's cells become less responsive to insulin, is often seen in women with PCOS. This leads to increased insulin production by the pancreas, which can disrupt the normal hormonal balance in the body.

Elevated levels of androgens, often referred to as "male hormones," are another characteristic of PCOS. These androgens, such as testosterone, can interfere with the development and release of eggs from the ovaries and can contribute to the formation of cysts. The precise mechanisms that lead to these hormonal imbalances are still being studied, but insulin resistance and increased insulin levels are believed to play a role.

Environmental Factors:

Certain environmental factors may contribute to the development of PCOS or exacerbate its symptoms. These factors include a sedentary lifestyle, poor dietary choices, exposure to endocrine-disrupting chemicals (EDCs), and stress.

Lack of physical activity and an unhealthy diet can contribute to insulin resistance and weight gain, both of which are associated with PCOS. Additionally, exposure to EDCs, which are chemicals found in many everyday products, including plastics, cosmetics, and pesticides, may disrupt the normal hormonal balance in the body and contribute to the development of PCOS.

Stress can also play a role in the development and progression of PCOS. Chronic stress can lead to elevated levels of cortisol, a stress hormone, which can disrupt the delicate hormonal balance in the body and contribute to insulin resistance and hormonal imbalances.

Other Factors:

Several other factors have been implicated in the origin of PCOS, although their exact contributions are still under investigation. These include prenatal androgen exposure, excess inflammation in the body, and alterations in gut microbiota.

Prenatal androgen exposure refers to high levels of androgens experienced by the foetus during pregnancy. This exposure may influence the development of the reproductive system and contribute to PCOS later in life.

Inflammation is believed to play a role in the development of PCOS. Chronic low-grade inflammation can disrupt normal hormone production and function, contributing to insulin resistance and hormonal imbalances.

Research has also suggested a possible link between alterations in gut microbiota, the community of microorganisms in the digestive tract, and PCOS. Disruptions in the balance of gut bacteria may impact hormonal regulation and metabolism, although further research is needed to fully understand this relationship.

In conclusion, the origin of PCOS is multifactorial, involving a complex interplay of genetic, hormonal, and environmental factors. Genetic predisposition, hormonal imbalances, such as insulin resistance and elevated androgens, environmental factors like sedentary lifestyle and exposure to endocrine-disrupting chemicals, as well as prenatal androgen exposure, inflammation, and alterations in gut microbiota, all contribute to the development and progression of PCOS. Understanding these factors is crucial for developing effective treatments and interventions to manage this condition.

**Chapter Four**

# WOMEN AND MENOPAUSE:

In the journey of life, women undergo numerous transformations that shape their physical, emotional, and mental well-being. Among these transformative phases, menopause holds a unique significance. It is a natural progression that marks the end of reproductive years, and although it may present various challenges, it also offers a gateway to self-discovery, empowerment, and an opportunity to embrace newfound freedom. In her captivating book, "Eternal Ecstasy: Ageless Sexual Bliss," esteemed author Dora J. Boye invites women to explore the extraordinary potential of menopause and embrace this transformative stage with confidence, grace, and a renewed sense of purpose.

Understanding Menopause:

Menopause is a natural biological process that occurs in women typically between the ages of 45 and 55. It signals the end of menstruation and the decline of reproductive hormones, particularly oestrogen and progesterone. While the physical symptoms can vary from woman to woman, common experiences include hot flashes, night sweats, mood swings, changes in libido, and vaginal dryness. However, it is important to recognize that menopause is not merely a collection of symptoms but a profound transition that affects women holistically.

Navigating Challenges:

With her insightful expertise, Dora J. Boye guides women through the challenges associated with menopause, offering practical advice and compassionate support. She encourages women to view this phase as an opportunity for self-care, self-discovery, and personal growth. By addressing the physical symptoms, such as through lifestyle adjustments, hormonal therapy, or alternative treatments, women can find relief and regain control over their bodies. Moreover, Boye highlights the importance of seeking emotional support, fostering healthy relationships, and practising self-compassion during this transformative period.

Unlocking Empowerment:

Contrary to popular belief, menopause is not the end of vitality and sensuality; rather, it opens doors to new possibilities. Dora J. Boye eloquently shares how menopause can be a time of self-realisation and empowerment. By embracing the changes in their bodies and minds, women can tap into a newfound wisdom and strength. Boye encourages women to explore their sexuality, redefining it based on their desires and preferences, and to embrace the ageless beauty that comes from inner contentment and self-confidence.

A Call to Women:

"Eternal Ecstasy: Ageless Sexual Bliss" serves as a rallying cry for women to view menopause as a transformative and empowering experience rather than a time of decline. Through her eloquent prose and compassionate guidance, Dora J. Boye empowers women to navigate this journey with grace and resilience, reminding them of their infinite potential. The book invites women of all backgrounds to join a community of support, celebrating the beauty and strength that menopause brings.

**Foot words.**

With "Eternal Ecstasy: Ageless Sexual Bliss," Dora J. Boye crafts an impressive narrative that captivates the attention of women seeking empowerment and self-discovery during the menopausal phase. By addressing the challenges, offering practical advice, and nurturing a sense of empowerment, Boye paves the way for women to embrace this transformative period with open hearts and minds. Through her words, women are encouraged to recognize the infinite possibilities that menopause presents, ultimately leading them to a state of eternal bliss and renewed vitality.

**Chapter Five**

# GREAT SEX NEVER GETS OLD

In the realm of human experience, there are few pleasures as profound and transformative as the intimate connection shared between two individuals. This connection transcends age, defying the constraints of time and reinforcing the notion that great sex truly never gets old. In the book "Eternal Ecstasy: Ageless Sexual Bliss," the author explores the timeless nature of sexual fulfilment, weaving a narrative that illustrates the enduring power of intimacy, desire, and passion. Through the author's personal journey, we discover that age is no barrier to experiencing profound ecstasy and unbridled pleasure.

Illustrative Story:

In the pages of "Eternal Ecstasy: Ageless Sexual Bliss," the author recounts their own remarkable journey to illustrate the central theme of the book. Let's delve into a story that encapsulates the essence of this transformative experience:

In their mid-60s, the author found themselves immersed in the societal belief that sexual satisfaction and passion diminish with age. Society often perpetuates the notion that the later stages of life are devoid of sensuality and that intimacy is reserved for the young. However, the author refused to accept this widely held belief, embarking on a personal quest to challenge these preconceptions.

One summer, during a retreat in a serene coastal town, the author encountered Muchalo, an intriguing man in his late 50s. Muchalo Exuded a magnetic aura, radiating confidence and sensuality. Over the course of their conversations, the author discovered that Muchalo embraced his sexuality and viewed it as a vital aspect of her well-being, irrespective of age.

Inspired by Muchalo's perspective, the author embarked on a transformative journey of self-discovery. They explored their own desires, challenged societal expectations, and embraced a newfound confidence in their sexuality. The author embarked on a journey of self-love, prioritising their physical and emotional well-being.

As the author's self-assurance grew, they experienced a profound shift in their intimate relationships. They discovered that age does not diminish desire, but rather enhances it with wisdom, experience, and a deeper appreciation for the intricacies of pleasure. The author's encounters with their partner became a symphony of touch, desire, and vulnerability, resulting in an unbounded sense of fulfilment and joy.

Through their personal journey, the author realised that great sex is not limited by age but is rather an eternal source of connection and self-expression. They understood that sexual bliss can be ageless, transcending the physical realm and enriching every aspect of life.

**Foot words:**

"Eternal Ecstasy: Ageless Sexual Bliss" is a testament to the enduring power of sexual fulfilment, transcending boundaries imposed by society and age. The author's story serves as an inspiring reminder that intimacy, desire, and passion can flourish at any stage of life. By embracing our own desires, challenging societal expectations, and nurturing a deeper understanding of ourselves, we can unlock the gateway to eternal sexual bliss. This book invites readers to embrace their own journey, unapologetically celebrating the timeless nature of great sex that truly never gets old.

## Chapter Six

# EARLY SYMPTOMS OF MENOPAUSE

Welcome to Chapter 6 of "Eternal Ecstasy: Ageless Sexual Bliss." In this chapter, we will explore the early symptoms of menopause, a natural phase that many women experience as they transition into a new stage of life. Understanding the signs and symptoms associated with menopause is essential for women to embrace their bodies' changes and navigate this transformative period with grace and confidence. By shedding light on this topic, we aim to empower our female readers to maintain their sexual well-being and embrace the joy of eternal ecstasy, irrespective of age. Understanding Menopause:

Menopause is a normal part of a woman's life cycle and usually occurs between the ages of 45 and 55. It marks the end of reproductive years and is characterised by the cessation of menstruation. However, before menstruation stops completely, women may experience a range of symptoms known as perimenopause.

Perimenopause:

Perimenopause refers to the transitional phase leading up to menopause. It can last for several years and is often marked by irregular menstrual cycles. During this time, women may experience various physical and emotional changes as their bodies adjust to hormonal fluctuations. Some common early symptoms of perimenopause include:

a. Irregular periods: Menstrual cycles may become shorter or longer, with heavier or lighter bleeding than usual.

b. Hot flashes: Sudden waves of heat that spread over the body, causing flushing and sweating.

c. Night sweats: Similar to hot flashes, but occurring primarily at night and interrupting sleep.

d. Vaginal dryness: Reduced natural lubrication, leading to discomfort or pain during sexual intercourse.

e. Mood swings: Fluctuating hormone levels can cause mood changes, including irritability, anxiety, and depression.

f. Sleep disturbances: Insomnia, waking up frequently during the night, or difficulty falling asleep.

g. Changes in libido: Some women may experience a decrease in sexual desire or changes in sexual responsiveness.

Managing Early Symptoms:

While the symptoms mentioned above can be challenging, it's important to remember that every woman's experience with menopause is unique. Here are some suggestions to help manage the early symptoms of menopause:

a. Stay informed: Educate yourself about menopause and its symptoms to better understand what you may be going through. Knowledge can empower you to make informed decisions regarding your health and well-being.

b. Communicate with your healthcare provider: Discuss your symptoms with a healthcare professional who can provide guidance, support, and potential treatment options tailored to your needs.

c. Adopt a healthy lifestyle: Regular exercise, a balanced diet, stress management techniques, and adequate sleep can help alleviate some menopausal symptoms.

d. Seek support: Connect with friends, support groups, or online communities to share experiences, gain advice, and find emotional support during this transformative time.

**Chapter Seven**

# MEN AND ANDROPAUSE

Facts about sexual health and vitality, men go through a natural ageing process that often accompanies changes in their hormone levels. While women experience menopause, men undergo a similar transition called andropause. "Eternal Ecstasy: Ageless Sexual Bliss" is a book that delves into the subject of andropause, helping men embrace this journey and maintain a fulfilling and blissful sexual life throughout their lives. This note aims to shed light on andropause, its early symptoms, and the importance of understanding them before buying into the concept of eternal sexual bliss. Understanding Andropause:

Andropause, sometimes referred to as "male menopause," is a gradual decline in testosterone levels that occurs in men as they age, typically starting in their late 40s or early 50s. Testosterone plays a crucial role in maintaining men's overall well-being, including sexual health, energy levels, muscle mass, and bone density. Although andropause is a natural and inevitable process, it can bring about various changes and challenges that affect a man's sexual satisfaction and overall quality of life.

Early Symptoms:

Recognizing the early symptoms of andropause is vital for men to seek appropriate guidance and support in managing this transition effectively. While the severity and onset of symptoms may vary among individuals, here are some common signs to be aware of:

Reduced Sexual Desire: A decline in libido or a decreased interest in sexual activity is often one of the first signs of andropause. Men may experience a shift in their sexual desires or find it more challenging to become aroused.

Erectile Dysfunction: Andropause can contribute to difficulties in achieving and maintaining erections. Men may notice a decrease in the firmness and frequency of their erections, leading to frustration and a decline in sexual confidence.

Fatigue and Reduced Energy Levels: As testosterone levels decline, men may experience persistent fatigue, reduced energy levels, and a lack of motivation. This can impact their sexual performance and overall enthusiasm for intimate activities.

Mood Changes: Hormonal fluctuations during andropause can lead to mood swings, irritability, anxiety, and even depression. These emotional changes may indirectly affect one's sexual well-being.

Changes in Body Composition: Andropause can result in a decrease in muscle mass, an increase in body fat, and a loss of overall strength. These physical changes can affect a man's body image and self-confidence, potentially impacting his sexual satisfaction.

The Importance of Understanding Symptoms:

"Eternal Ecstasy: Ageless Sexual Bliss" emphasises the significance of understanding andropause symptoms before embarking on any potential remedies or treatments. By being aware of the early signs, men can take proactive steps toward managing andropause effectively. Seeking medical advice, adopting a healthy lifestyle, maintaining open communication with partners, and exploring potential therapies can contribute to a more fulfilling and blissful sexual life, even during andropause.

**Foot words**

In the journey of eternal sexual bliss, it is crucial to embrace the realities of andropause and recognize its early symptoms. "Eternal Ecstasy: Ageless Sexual Bliss" serves as a guide, providing men with the knowledge and understanding they need to navigate the challenges of andropause. By empowering men to proactively address these changes and seek appropriate support, this book aims to help them maintain a fulfilling, satisfying, and blissful sexual life at every stage of their lives.

## Chapter Eight

# THE UGLY QUESTION PART 1

**Do we lose our hormones because we age?**

It is not uncommon for individuals to wonder about the role of hormones as we age. Many popular notions suggest that ageing inevitably leads to a decline in hormones, ultimately dampening our sexual vitality and pleasure. However, it is crucial to critically examine this belief and dispel any misconceptions that may hinder our pursuit of lifelong satisfaction and fulfilment.

Understanding Hormones and Aging:

Hormones are chemical messengers produced by the endocrine glands that regulate various bodily functions, including sexual desire, reproduction, and overall well-being. It is true that hormone levels naturally fluctuate throughout our lives, with some declining as we age. However, the notion that we completely lose our hormones as we grow older is a misinterpretation of the complex relationship between hormones and ageing.

Hormonal Changes in Aging:

As we age, certain hormones do exhibit changes in their production and regulation. For instance, women experience menopause, a natural transition marked by a decline in oestrogen and progesterone levels, resulting in various physical and emotional changes. Similarly, men may experience andropause, often characterised by a gradual decline in testosterone levels. These hormonal shifts can affect sexual desire, arousal, and overall sexual function.

However, it is important to note that not all individuals experience the same degree of hormonal changes, and the impact of these changes varies significantly from person to person. Furthermore, other factors, such as lifestyle, overall health, and psychological well-being, play a significant role in determining sexual satisfaction and pleasure, regardless of hormonal fluctuations.

The Influence of Lifestyle Factors:

Maintaining a healthy lifestyle is crucial for nurturing sexual well-being and satisfaction throughout our lives. Regular exercise, a balanced diet, adequate sleep, and stress management all contribute to overall vitality and sexual health. These lifestyle factors can positively influence hormone levels and sexual function, helping individuals experience a more fulfilling and joyful sexual life, even as they age.

The Power of Psychological Well-being:

Psychological factors play a significant role in sexual satisfaction, irrespective of hormonal changes. Emotional intimacy, communication, self-esteem, and body image are critical components of a fulfilling sexual relationship. Maintaining healthy mental well-being and nurturing positive attitudes towards ageing can enhance sexual pleasure and ensure an enduring sense of ecstasy throughout our lives.

Seeking Professional Support:

If individuals experience significant disruptions in sexual desire or function due to hormonal changes, seeking professional medical advice is recommended. Healthcare providers can offer appropriate guidance, including hormone replacement therapy or other interventions, to help individuals address specific concerns and optimise their sexual well-being.

**Foot words**

In the pursuit of eternal ecstasy and ageless sexual bliss, it is essential to dispel the myth that we inevitably lose our hormones as we age. While hormonal changes can occur, they do not equate to a complete loss of sexual vitality. By focusing on healthy lifestyle choices, nurturing psychological well-being, and seeking professional support when necessary, individuals can continue to experience sexual pleasure and satisfaction throughout their lives. Embracing a holistic approach to sexual well-being enables us to age gracefully, embracing the joy and ecstasy of intimate connections at any stage of life.

## Chapter Nine

# THE UGLY QUESTION PART 2

**Do we age because we lose our hormones?**

In the pursuit of eternal youth and boundless pleasure, the connection between hormones and ageing has sparked considerable interest. The book, "Eternal Ecstasy: Ageless Sexual Bliss," delves into this intriguing topic, exploring the impact of hormones on the ageing process and how it relates to maintaining a fulfilling and vibrant sexual life. By unravelling the secrets behind hormone regulation, this book aims to captivate readers and guide them towards achieving a timeless state of ecstasy and ageless vitality.

Understanding Hormones and Aging:

Hormones play a vital role in our overall health and well-being, including the ageing process. As we grow older, hormonal levels tend to decline, leading to various physiological changes. However, it is essential to note that ageing itself is a complex process influenced by multiple factors, including genetics, lifestyle, and environmental elements.

The Influence of Hormones on Sexual Bliss:

One area where hormones significantly impact our lives is in the realm of sexual well-being. Hormones, such as oestrogen, testosterone, progesterone, and others, influence libido, arousal, and overall sexual function. As we age, the decline in these hormones can lead to a decrease in sexual desire, diminished sexual response, and changes in sexual satisfaction.

Unveiling the Secrets:

"Eternal Ecstasy: Ageless Sexual Bliss" delves deep into the mechanisms of hormones and ageing, shedding light on how individuals can maintain their vitality and sexual bliss despite the natural decline in hormone levels. Through a comprehensive exploration of hormone replacement therapies, lifestyle modifications, and other cutting-edge approaches, the book provides readers with practical tools to enhance their sexual well-being and overall satisfaction.

Navigating the Path to Ageless Sexual Bliss:

The book offers a holistic approach to achieving ageless sexual bliss by addressing various facets of life that influence hormonal balance and sexual vitality. It guides readers through the following key areas:

Hormone Optimization: Discussing the role of hormone replacement therapy, natural remedies, and lifestyle choices in promoting hormonal balance and rejuvenation.

Nutrition and Exercise: Highlighting the significance of a balanced diet and regular physical activity in supporting hormone production and overall well-being.

Emotional and Mental Well-being: Exploring the psychological aspects of sexual bliss, including the importance of self-love, stress reduction techniques, and maintaining healthy relationships.

Lifestyle Choices: Discussing the impact of factors like sleep, environmental toxins, and personal habits on hormonal health and sexual satisfaction.

**Chapter Ten**

# MOOD CHANGES

We live in a world where our emotions and moods shape our experiences and define our well-being. As human beings, we constantly seek ways to enhance our happiness and find fulfilment in various aspects of life. One of the most profound and transformative areas where mood changes can significantly impact our lives is in the realm of sexuality. It is with great pleasure that I present to you "Eternal Ecstasy: Ageless Sexual Bliss," a book that delves deep into the exploration of mood changes and their potential to elevate our sexual experiences to unprecedented heights.

Within the pages of this extraordinary book, you will embark on a journey of self-discovery and empowerment. Drawing from a wealth of scientific research and practical wisdom, "Eternal Ecstasy: Ageless Sexual Bliss" reveals the keys to unlocking the immense potential that lies within your own mood fluctuations. This book is designed to impress upon you the profound impact your moods can have on your sexual encounters, and how you can harness this power to create a truly fulfilling and blissful experience.

Through the expert guidance of renowned psychologists, sexologists, and relationship experts, you will gain invaluable insights into the intricate connections between our emotional states and sexual well-being. You will learn to identify and embrace the full spectrum of your moods, understanding how each one can be a gateway to profound pleasure and intimacy. From the passionate intensity of desire to the tender vulnerability of love, this book will guide you in navigating the myriad emotional landscapes that make up the tapestry of human sexuality.

Furthermore, "Eternal Ecstasy: Ageless Sexual Bliss" goes beyond the conventional approaches to pleasure and arousal. It explores holistic practices, mindful techniques, and cutting-edge research to help you expand your awareness and tap into the limitless possibilities that lie within your own being. With practical exercises and thought-provoking reflections, you will embark on a personal transformation that will not only enhance your sexual experiences but also enrich your entire existence.

The power of this book lies not only in its profound insights but also in its ability to inspire and empower. As you read its pages, you will feel a renewed sense of excitement and curiosity, eager to explore the depths of your own desires and emotions. The knowledge and wisdom contained within "Eternal Ecstasy:

Ageless Sexual Bliss" will become a trusted companion on your journey to lifelong sexual fulfilment.

In conclusion, "Eternal Ecstasy: Ageless Sexual Bliss" is a masterpiece that brings together the realms of mood changes and sexual bliss, offering you a profound understanding of the transformative potential that lies within. Prepare to embark on an adventure of self-discovery, where you will embrace your moods and unlock the door to eternal ecstasy. It is my sincere hope that this book will not only impress but also empower you to embrace your sexuality fully and experience a lifetime of ageless sexual bliss.

# CONCLUSION

" Ageless Sexual Bliss" is a provocative and enlightening book that explores the concept of eternal pleasure and ageless sexual fulfilment. Authored by an expert in human sexuality and spiritual exploration, the book delves into the realms of pleasure, desire, and the potential for transformative sexual experiences that transcend the boundaries of time.

The central theme of the book revolves around the belief that sexual pleasure has the potential to be an eternal and transcendent experience, defying the limitations of age and societal norms. It challenges conventional notions of sexuality, inviting readers to explore the possibilities of a deeper connection with their own sexual desires and the transformative power that can be harnessed through them.

The book offers a comprehensive analysis of various perspectives on sexuality, drawing from ancient wisdom, spiritual practices, and modern research. It delves into the teachings of ancient cultures that viewed sexuality as a sacred and spiritual experience, emphasising the importance of cultivating a harmonious relationship between body, mind, and spirit.

Through the exploration of various practices, including tantric traditions, meditation, and mindfulness, the book provides practical guidance on how individuals can tap into their sexual energy to achieve profound states of pleasure and fulfilment. It encourages readers to embrace their unique desires and preferences, free from societal constraints, and to embark on a journey of self-discovery and sexual liberation.

Furthermore, "Eternal Ecstasy: Ageless Sexual Bliss" explores the concept of agelessness in sexual experiences. It challenges the notion that sexual pleasure diminishes with age, presenting a compelling argument for the continued exploration and cultivation of sexual satisfaction throughout one's lifetime. The book introduces techniques and strategies for maintaining and enhancing sexual intimacy as individuals age, promoting a positive and empowering perspective on sexuality in later stages of life.

Importantly, the book emphasises the importance of consent, respect, and ethical behaviour in sexual encounters. It addresses issues such as communication, boundaries, and the necessity of creating safe and consensual environments for sexual exploration.

In conclusion, "Eternal Ecstasy: Ageless Sexual Bliss" is a thought-provoking book that delves into the realms of pleasure, desire, and the potential for transformative sexual experiences. It challenges societal norms, encouraging readers to embrace their unique sexual desires and cultivate a harmonious relationship with their bodies and spirits. By drawing from ancient wisdom and modern research, the book provides practical guidance for individuals seeking to tap into their sexual energy and achieve ageless sexual fulfilment. Ultimately, it serves as an invitation to explore the depths of human sexuality and discover the potential for eternal pleasure and bliss.